Table of Contents

INTRODUCTION

Nearly 300,000 people are admitted to the hospital for pancreatitis each year in the United States. This is a very serious and painful condition that requires careful medical observation. In fact, during the first few days, no food or liquid is allowed; all fluids are administered through an IV.

As the pancreas begins to heal and function once again, first clear liquids are allowed and then bland, low-fat foods are added under the watchful eye of the health care team to make sure that food is well-tolerated. Acute pancreatitis can be life-threatening; seeking medical treatment is a must.

While the majority of people will recover well from acute pancreatitis, nearly 25 percent of those diagnosed will experience recurrent episodes, leading the disease to become chronic. Chronic pancreatitis puts you at a significantly increased risk of developing pancreatic cancer, diabetes, liver failure and other potentially life-threatening illnesses.

Not only is following a diet for pancreatitis necessary to help recover, but it is essential to help prevent this disease from entering the chronic phase. There are some individuals who are more prone to developing pancreatitis, including those with a history of substance abuse, use of certain prescription drugs, unhealthy eating and genetics.

Light-to-moderate exercise, yoga and meditation can help manage the symptoms and avoiding alcohol and tobacco are absolutely necessary for recovery. Whether you've been recently diagnosed with acute pancreatitis or chronic pancreatitis, the first step is adopting a healthy diet focusing on fresh fruits and vegetables, whole grains and lean proteins.

The Pancreas Diet is found in the book. The Pancreatic diet cookbook by Emily green RND, a registered nurse, social worker and health counselor.

She says that this is not a diet book, or a book for diabetics but instead is a healthy eating lifestyle guide for everyone.

In this book Emily explains how eating the right foods can protect your pancreas and promote health, whereas when you eat unhealthy foods you are abusing your pancreas. By following the guidelines outlined in this program you will be able to discover the foods that help your pancreas function optimally so that you can easily lose weight.

Pancreas Diet Basics

In The Pancreatic diet cookbook readers learn about the connection between a healthy pancreas and long-term wellbeing. Green believes that "pancreatic abuse" is a major risk factor for the development of a number of chronic diseases – not just diabetes – including conditions such as heart disease, stroke, high blood pressure, kidney problems, and polycystic ovarian syndrome.

The goal of the program is to reduce the workload on your pancreas by learning which foods keep your blood sugar in balance. This is achieved by monitoring your blood glucose levels four to six times each day after eating and recording the results in comparison with your food selections.

The diet does not require any calorie or carbohydrate counting but it is necessary to eliminate all foods containing sugar as well as high glycemic carbohydrates like bread, potatoes, rice and pasta. Artificial sweeteners must be strictly avoided and alcohol intake should be limited or eliminated entirely.

Fruit is permitted in moderate amounts, however, it must always be eaten alone (with two exceptions: apples with almond butter and Candice's Super Smoothie). You should emphasize green vegetables and plant-based proteins such as tofu, tempeh and legumes, while limiting animal protein and avoiding dairy products.

An eating pattern involving five hours between meals is recommended but in the beginning you may need snacks as your body and pancreas adjusts to a new way of eating.

Dieters are advised to use a rather long list of nutritional supplements including multivitamins and minerals, coenzyme Q10 and fish oil. Emily clearly explains the purpose of each of the recommended products and outlines how they work to improve your health.

Pancreatitis Diet

After a diagnosis of acute or chronic pancreatitis, nutrition must be the first priority. The goal with a pancreatitis diet is to prevent malnutrition, nutritional deficiencies and optimize blood sugar levels while protecting against kidney and liver problems, pancreatic cancer and worsening symptoms. Columbia University's Pancreas Center recommends focusing on a nutrient-dense diet high in lean proteins, whole grains, fruits, vegetables and low-fat dairy products while avoiding greasy fried foods and alcohol. Their program recommends annual blood tests to determine any nutrient deficiencies and recommends supplementation as necessary. The diet recommended by Columbia University is very similar to the Mediterranean diet followed for generations throughout Greece, Italy and Spain. Countless studies have found that this way of eating helps to lower the risk of Type 2 diabetes; improves A1C levels; improves cognition and elevates mood; protects against Alzheimer's disease and heart disease; protects against many gastrointestinal cancers and is associated with lower a lower risk of pancreatic cancer.

The traditional Mediterranean diet may be a touch too high in fats for some individuals with pancreatitis, but it is easily modified. Yes, even healthy fats like olive oil, coconut oil and those from wild-caught fish and grass-fed meats can be too intense for some with this condition. Like so many other diseases, the first step has to be listening to your body and recognizing the foods that make you feel at your best.

The majority of each meal should focus on fruits, vegetables and whole grains with proteins and fats playing a supporting role. Many experts support the following daily servings as a target:

- 3 servings of whole grains
- 2 servings of fresh fruit
- 5–7 servings of vegetables
- 1 serving of nuts
- 1 serving of lean animal protein
- 1 serving of low-fat dairy

Weekly:

- 3 servings of wild-caught fish
- No more than 2 servings of beef or lamb
- 3 servings of eggs
- 3–4 servings of chicken or turkey
- 3–4 servings of nuts or seeds
- 1–2 servings of heart-healthy sweets

- 4–6 servings of legumes

The real goal here is to provide the body with foods that are easy to digest and that don't cause the blood sugar to spike, while also keeping you satisfied. It is important to eat foods to address any nutritional deficiencies that pancreatitis may be causing. Remember, this is a guideline. If you have pancreatitis and there are foods on this list that you know you are allergic or sensitive to, please avoid them.

Top 8 Fruits

Blackberries and blueberries: These berries are rich in resveratrol, manganese, fiber and vitamins C and K, which support healthy digestion while fighting cancer. Try this bright and nutrient-dense Blackberry Lemon Salad that features heart-healthy olive oil, sesame seeds and almonds.

Cherries: Low in calories and high in essential nutrients, cherries are a perfect snack that supports weight loss, reduces inflammation and promotes restful sleep.

Watermelon: Excellent source of vitamins A, B and C as well as potassium, magnesium and manganese. Have a watermelon smoothie for breakfast or an afternoon snack; the protein in this recipe comes from coconut yogurt and chia seeds.

Black plums: With a low glycemic index, plus proven to lower cholesterol and aid in digestion, plums are a perfect fruit to eat on a pancreatitis diet.

Red grapes: The polyphenols in grapes have been shown to help prevent obesity and Type 2 diabetes while lowering inflammation. To incorporate them into your diet, and reap the help benefits, have a handful as a snack or try this satisfying grape, chicken, and walnut salad.

Mangos: With healthy fiber and vitamin C, mangos also contain essential minerals, including iron, calcium, potassium and magnesium. This super fruit is associated with improved blood glucose levels and glycemic control. As an occasional sweet treat, try this amazing Mango Coconut Ice Cream, which gets its richness from egg yolks and coconut milk and its sweetness from raw honey and the mangos.

Apples: Because they are naturally high in fiber, help lower inflammation and aid in digestion, apples make a quick, healthy snack. As a side dish or dessert, this Baked Quinoa and Apple dish is both warming and satisfying, while also supplying protein and healthy fiber.

Pomegranate: Sweet and crunchy, this super fruit is loaded with fiber, potassium and vitamins C and K. Take a handful and toss them on top of protein-rich hummus as they do in many areas of the Middle East.

Top 7 Vegetables:

Beets: Packed with essential nutrients like iron, manganese, copper, potassium and the B vitamins, beets are known to improve heart health, brain health and support liver function. Try this family-friendly Roasted Beets with Balsamic Glaze alongside your favorite lean protein.

Broccoli: Just a cup of cooked broccoli contains more than 100 percent of one's daily value of both vitamin K and vitamin C. Also rich with minerals, this vegetable fights cancer and promotes digestive health. For a satisfying meal, try my recipe for Alfredo Chicken and Broccoli Casserole, featuring whole grain pasta, lean chicken, kefir and aged cheese. (17)

Spinach: Popeye wasn't wrong; spinach is packed with nutrients that boost immunity, protect against diabetes and protect against certain types of cancer. Try this Mango Walnut Spinach Salad, which combines many foods on the pancreatitis diet list.

Kale: A cruciferous vegetable that demonstrates anti-inflammatory properties, supports detoxification, eye health, and protects against cancer, kale is a nutrient-dense leafy green perfect for any diet for pancreatitis. Add a few leaves to a smoothie or replace some (or all!) lettuce in a salad with finely chopped kale.

Lettuce: Salads are a big part of a Mediterranean diet and an easy way to ensure you meet the recommended five to seven servings of vegetables each day. Choose darker leaf lettuces and mixed wild greens to enjoy the highest levels of vitamins and minerals.

Sweet potatoes: Rich with beta carotene, vitamin C, copper, vitamin B6, and manganese, sweet potatoes are a healthy starch that tastes great. In the mornings, alongside a couple of cage-free eggs, this Sweet Potato Hash Brown recipe will leave you energized for the day.

Carrots: Beta carotene is associated with immune system health and eye health, as well as healthy digestion, while being one of the most versatile vegetables on the planet. Enjoy carrots raw, cooked or juiced on your pancreatitis diet.

Top 6 Whole Grains:

Research shows that whole grains in a pancreatic diet should be encouraged.

Brown rice: High in fiber and rich in manganese, replacing white rice with brown rice can lower your risk for Type 2 diabetes by 16 percent. As a side dish, this gluten-free grain is relatively high in calories, so sticking with a single serving size is recommended.

Buckwheat: High in protein and fiber, this gluten-free grain is rich in antioxidants and is highly digestible. Buckwheat flour can be used for making a healthy morning pancake, while buckwheat groats can be added to salads or made into a morning porridge.

Polenta: This rough grind of corn, similar to Southern grits, is used throughout the Mediterranean. Top it with mushrooms and legumes, a touch of feta cheese, and fresh herbs for a filling and satiating meal. Purchase organic, non-GMO polenta only.

Millet: High in fiber, naturally gluten-free and easy to digest, millet is a seed, often misrepresented as a grain. This nutrient-dense seed is experiencing a renaissance because it is so very versatile. Explore millet recipes suitable for breakfast, lunch and dinner

Teff: If you aren't familiar with the Ethiopian grain teff, it's time to introduce yourself. This grain promotes weight loss, boosts the immune system, supports bone health and aids in digestion. It's available as a flour or grain, and you can use it to make porridges, pancakes and tortillas.

Amaranth: Prized for thousands of years by the Aztecs, this grain is a great source of fiber, manganese and protein. This gluten-free whole grain aids in digestive health, reduces inflammation, fights the development of Type 2 diabetes and aids in weight loss. Use in place of oats, white rice or pasta, and as a thickener for soups.

Top 5 Nuts and Seeds:

Almonds: A distant relative of many stone fruits, the simple almond is packed with protein, fiber and a host of essential vitamins and minerals. Research shows they help to control blood sugar levels, help with weight loss and may increase nutrient absorption of fat-soluble nutrients. Because of their relatively high-fat content, limit yourself to a single serving.

Walnuts: A real nutrient powerhouse, walnuts provide omega-3s, supporting a healthy heart and brain while helping to control inflammation and blood sugar levels. For an occasional healthy sweet treat, try my recipe for Raw Brownie Bites, which features walnuts, almonds, cacao powder and dates.

Sunflower seeds: Rich in the B vitamins and vitamin E as well as selenium and magnesium, sunflower seeds provide a healthy dose of essential fatty acids, amino acids and fiber. Eat in moderation, and stick to a half of a single serving as their fat content is relatively high.

Pumpkin seeds: Once only a fall snack, pumpkin seeds are now available year-round. With a satisfying crunch, and packed with healthy fats, protein and fiber, pumpkin seeds are tasty tossed on salads or enjoyed mixed into yogurt. As a snack, it's hard to beat this recipe for Spicy Roasted Pumpkin Seeds.

Pistachios: Grown throughout the Mediterranean, it is no surprise that pistachios make this list. They are known to help lower cholesterol and help with weight loss. Stick with one-half of an ounce as a serving due to the fat content. While they are great in pilafs and salads, it's hard to beat a handful of pistachios for a quick burst of energy.

Top 4 Lean Protein Sources:

Wild-caught fish: The typical Mediterranean diets feature a wild-caught fish or seafood at least twice each week. Wild-caught salmon is associated with healthy cognitive function, heart health and cancer protection.

Poultry: Lean cuts of chicken and turkey are a great source of protein. Stick with grilling, baking or poaching – avoid frying to keep the fat content within healthy levels. And to help with digestion, consume chicken bone broth that is naturally rich with collagen and L-glutamine, which is shown to preserve gut integrity while altering gut microbiota (flora) to improve digestive functioning.

Eggs: Cage-free eggs are high in protein, rich in amino acids and have less saturated fat than their counterparts. Eggs, a typical breakfast staple, are also great for quick lunches and dinners. Pancakes for dinner? Sure, when they are Banana Egg Paleo Pancakes, why not!

Legumes: High in protein, low in fat and high in fiber, legumes are an essential part of a healthy pancreatitis diet as they help to stabilize blood sugar levels and aid in weight loss. Specific beans including lentils, mung beans and garbanzo beans contain lipase, a digestive enzyme released by the pancreas. Try adding a variety of beans to your diet with hummus for lunch or a bowl of stick-to-your-ribs, Turkey Chili with Adzuki Beans.

Top 3 Low-Fat Dairy:

Greek yogurt: Choose fat-free or low-fat Greek yogurt without added sugar or sweeteners while following a pancreatitis diet. High in probiotics for gut health and protein, this dairy product is perfect for breakfast when partnered with a whole grain toast and berries.

Cottage cheese: Rich in vitamin B12 and high in calcium, cottage cheese is a great snack, particularly when partnered with other foods from the pancreatitis diet list like nuts, seeds and fruit.

Kefir: Known for its immunity-boosting powers and healthy bacteria, which aids in digestion, this cultured dairy product provides protein, calcium and vitamin D.

Enjoy kefir as a mid-morning snack, or use it in place of another dairy in your favorite smoothie.

Alcohol, tobacco and caffeine

Known or suspected allergens like wheat, soy, dairy, corn and artificial sweeteners

Fried foods

White flour products like pasta and white bread

Sugar

Trans-fatty acids in commercially-prepared foods

Lifestyle Changes to Prevent Pancreatitis Recurrence

If you smoke cigarettes or use other tobacco products, stop.

Eat three to four small meals each day.

Stay hydrated; drink at least 8 ounces of water per 10 pounds of body weight each day.

Meditate and practice relaxation to ease stress and pain.

Practice yoga twice each week. According to a study published in the World Journal of Gastroenterology, yoga improves overall quality of life for those with chronic pancreatitis.

What are the Different Types of Pancreatic Diet

Different types of pancreatic diet plans include those that are meant to reduce the risk of a particular disease or condition and those that are meant to help with the recovery of a pancreatic illness. The main type of disease that afflicts the pancreas is pancreatic cancer, and it remains one of the leading causes of cancer death because it does not respond well to current treatment options. A diet used to prevent pancreatic cancer is generally low in calories to allow patients to lose or avoid gaining weight. Treatment diets for cancer patients and those with other diseases of the pancreas are usually heavily restricted.

Research has indicated that obesity is one of the main risk factors for developing pancreatic cancer. Not only does it put more strain on every organ in the body to carry around so much extra body weight, but it also increases the production of a protein called the Insulin-Like Growth Factor (IGF). IGF has been linked to an increase in lesions on the pancreas, a known cause of pancreatic cancer. By restricting calories, much lower levels of IGF are produced and lesions may not form.

Most different types of pancreatic diet plans are very low in fat and are also low in calories. Those who are trying to prevent the growth of lesions and pancreatic cancer cells should limit fat intake, primarily that coming from red meat and whole dairy. While the link between obesity and pancreatic cancer is still not entirely understood, controlling weight is known to help reduce the risk of nearly all types of cancer. Dieters with no known risk factors for pancreatic cancer should eat low-fat foods, although the occasional fatty food is generally acceptable.

Patients who are recovering from surgery of the pancreas or from pancreatic cancer treatments should slowly incorporate foods into the diet. There are different types of pancreatic diet plans for current patients, but they are mostly similar in that for the first several days, only water and broths are permitted. Afterward, things like toast, honey, coffee, soup, and tea can be added. Even more slowly, vegetables and then fats are added back into the diet.

Anyone who has a history of pancreatic cancer or disease should consult a physician before starting any type of the many different types of pancreatic diet plans. Although a low calorie diet is generally considered safe for most people, it is a good idea to determine any risk factors and conditions before food is heavily restricted. Those who are already at a healthy weight should simply cut back on red meat and other highly fattening foods and load up on more vegetables, especially those with antioxidants and other cancer fighting agents.

Best foods to eat for pancreatitis

Beans and lentils may be recommended for a pancreatitis diet because of their high fiber content. The first treatment for pancreatitis sometimes requires a person to refrain from consuming all food and liquids for several hours or even days.

Some people may need an alternate way of getting nutrition if they are unable to consume the required amounts for their body to work properly. When a doctor allows a person to eat again, they will likely recommend that a person eats small meals frequently throughout the day and avoids fast food, fried foods, and highly processed foods.

Here is a list of foods that may be recommended and why:

- vegetables
- beans and lentils
- fruits
- whole grains
- other plant-based foods that are not fried

These foods are recommended for people with pancreatitis because they tend to be naturally low in fat, which eases the amount of work the pancreas needs to do to aid digestion.

Fruits, vegetables, beans, lentils, and whole grains are also beneficial because of their fiber content. Eating more fiber can lower the chances of having gallstones or elevated levels of fats in the blood called triglycerides. Both of those conditions are common causes of acute pancreatitis.

In addition to fiber, the foods listed above also provide antioxidants. Pancreatitis is an inflammatory condition, and antioxidants may help reduce inflammation.

Lean meats

Lean meats can help people with pancreatitis meet their protein needs.

Medium-chain triglycerides (MCTs)

For people with chronic pancreatitis, adding MCTs to their diet may improve nutrient absorption. People often consume MCTs in supplement form as MCT oil. This supplement is available online without a prescription.

List of foods to avoid with pancreatitis
Alcohol may increase the risk of chronic pancreatitis and should be avoided.

Alcohol

Drinking alcohol during an acute pancreatitis attack can worsen the condition or contribute to chronic pancreatitis. Chronic alcohol use can also cause high triglyceride levels, a major risk factor for pancreatitis. For people whose chronic pancreatitis is caused by alcohol abuse, drinking alcohol can result in severe health issues and even death.

Fried foods and high-fat foods

Fried foods and high-fat foods, such as burgers and french fries, can be problematic for people with pancreatitis. The pancreas helps with fat digestion, so foods with more fat make the pancreas work harder.

Other examples of high-fat foods to avoid, include:

dairy products

processed meats, such as hot dogs and sausage

mayonnaise

potato chips

Eating these types of processed, high-fat foods can also lead to heart disease.

Refined carbohydrates

Registered dietitian Deborah Gerszberg recommends that people with chronic pancreatitis limit their intake of refined carbohydrates, such as white bread and high sugar foods. Refined carbohydrates can lead to the pancreas releasing larger amounts of insulin.

Foods that are high in sugar can also raise triglycerides. High triglyceride levels are a risk factor for acute pancreatitis.

Diet tips for recovering from pancreatitis

People recovering from pancreatitis may find that they tolerate smaller, more frequent meals. Eating six times per day may work better than eating three meals per day. A moderate fat diet, providing around 25 percent of calories from fat, may be tolerated by many people with chronic pancreatitis. The Cleveland Clinic recommend that people recovering from acute pancreatitis eat less than 30 grams of fat per day.

Prevention tips

Certain risk factors for pancreatitis, such as family history, cannot be changed. However, people can change some lifestyle factors that impact risk.

Obesity increases the risk for pancreatitis, so achieving and maintaining a healthy weight may help lower risk of developing pancreatitis. A healthy weight also lowers risk for gallstones, which are a common cause of pancreatitis.

Drinking large amounts of alcohol and smoking also raise an individual's risk for pancreatitis, so cutting back or avoiding these can help with preventing the condition.

Other treatment options

Vitamin supplements may be recommended, and the type of vitamin will depend on the individual.

Treatment for pancreatitis may involve hospitalization, intravenous fluids, pain medicine, and antibiotics. A doctor may prescribe a low-fat diet, but people who are unable to eat by mouth may need an alternate way of receiving nutrition. Surgery or other medical procedures may be recommended for some cases of pancreatitis.

People with chronic pancreatitis may have difficulty digesting and absorbing certain nutrients. These issues raise the risk of the person becoming malnourished. People with chronic pancreatitis may need to take digestive enzyme pills to help with digestion and absorbing nutrients.

Depending on the person, certain vitamin supplements may be recommended. Supplements may include the following:

- multivitamin
- calcium
- iron
- folate
- vitamin A
- vitamin D
- vitamin E
- vitamin K

- vitamin B-12

People should ask their healthcare provider if they should take a multivitamin. Consuming adequate amounts of fluid is also important. It is also important to speak to a healthcare provider before starting to take any supplements, such as MCT oil.

Pancreatic Liquid Diet

After the pancreas has cooled down and the pain faded then the next step will probably be to use a pancreatic liquid diet to slowly reintroduce you to food. The diet that you will be prescribed are usually called a clear liquids diet and a full liquids diet. The idea that Doctors use is that food needs to be introduced slowly to allow the pancreas to slowly start full functioning again.

Clear Pancreatic Liquid Diet

Clear liquids will generally be introduced first then if the pancreatitis tolerates this well either a full liquid diet or a solid diet will be prescribed. Clear Liquids are described as those that can be seen through. These liquids are more easily absorbed by the intestines and cause less stress to the pancreas.

Even though they contain some nutrition they are incapable of meeting the bodies energy requirements for more than a couple of days. This type of diet would include things like:

Bouillon soup without vegetables or noodles.

Coffee.

Fruit juices without pulp.

Gelatin

Popsicles

Soft drinks

Sports drinks

Tea

Water

After several days or more recovering from an attack of Pancreatitis it's amazing how good even gelatin can taste. It's almost like your taste buds have been reset and are tasting the food you are eating anew.

Full Pancreatic Liquid Diet

In some cases after you tolerate a pancreatic clear liquid diet instead of allowing a person to start a solid diet Doctors will want to have you try a full liquid diet. These pancreatic liquid diets include everything in a clear liquid diet but also include:

Cream of wheat

Fruit juices with pulp

Honey

Jelly

Milk, milkshakes and ice cream

Nutrition supplement drinks like Ensure or Boost

Pureed meats or vegetables

Soups with only a few solids

Vegetable juices

Yogurt and pudding

Pancreatitis Diet Recipes

Pancreaitis diet recipes is a brand new category and my hope is that you'll find it to be helpful in your journey to better health.

Most pancreatitis diet recipes you can find on the internet are not safe. They are conjured up by those who really don't know what can be eaten in relative safety and what foods should never be eaten.

When coming out of an acute attack I've heard of people being fed or told they can eat some of the most dangerous foods, by hospital employees (doctors, nutritionists, etc). Those who suffer from chronic disease have no real guidance. They have no guidance because, let's face the truth, you are worth more sick than welf you're well you don't visit the hospital ER rooms. You don't need routine office visits. You don't need prescription drugs or surgical procedures.

It is absolutely amazing to me how little the medical profession knows or is willing to tell about what is safe and what isn't safe for pancreatitis patient to eat. This holds true for nutritionists as well. As a result ... Safe pancreatitis diet recipes are extremely hard to find.

This new book category will endeavor to bring you a variety of decent tasting foods you will be able to enjoy in relative safety. Remember ... If you are still experiencing symptoms because you have not healed it is best to eat what I have termed as a modified vegan meal plan.

The Modified Vegan
Modified vegan simply means your food comes from plant sources, not animal sources. True vegans do not eat animal products however ... They do eat foods that you and I should not. Just because something grows in the ground or on a bush or tree which grows in the ground doesn't mean it is safe. If you haven't read my post on

pancreatitis diet basics you should do that. You should also read all the other posts about diet.

Vegans eat high fat foods such as nuts and seeds. Nuts and seeds are not safe. They eat and use oils in cooking. Oils are not safe. They eat avocado, coconut, soybeans and soy products which are not safe. Not for those of us who suffer with pancreatitis.

Once you have healed enough to be symptom free you can then begin to explore the short list of relatively safe animal foods. Now ... IF you have had only one mild attack and there isn't a lot of damage or an underlying cause that hasn't been addressed (be advised a pancreas doesn't simply wake up one morning and decide to become inflamed) you have an extremely good chance of healing totally, never having to worry about chronic disease but...

IF you are suffering from chronic pancreatitis or you have had more than one or two acute pancreatitis attacks and have not yet been diagnosed with chronic pancreatitis (even though you have ongoing, unrelenting symptoms) I would highly suggest the first place to start should be to begin a food diary.

You will quickly note that this section is a little premature if you really want to learn what you should and should NOT eat. Rather than take my word for it doing a proper food diary is the ONLY way you can learn what foods work for you and what foods do not work for you. Then ... This section containing pancreatitis diet recipes will become a valuable resource

Pancreatitis recipes

Oil Free Salad Dressings

Oil free salad dressings can be a tasty treat for those who need to avoid oil consumption. The following salad dressings are oil free and perfect for people like us (pancreatitis patients). Salads are great for those who have pancreatitis.

Salads (greens and other veggies) are safe food. Salads are full of vegetables (leafy greens, cruciferous, tubers, legumes, etc) which contain tons of essential nutrients, minerals and antioxidants (phytonutrients).

The problem with salads is that they taste somewhat bland to awful without something to dress them up and add that taste bud anticipation. And that is where good oil free salad dressings shine.

You'll need a clear shaker cup. If you don't have a clear one any kind of shaker cup will do. You could even mix the ingredients with a spoon, cup or small bowl if you don't have a shaker cup. Whatever works!

Once you have your dressing made you can either drizzle dressing onto your salad or you can dump the dressing on the salad (in a bowl) and toss it till it's all mixed. Whatever works for you.

The following dressings are my favorites but you can vary any of them in any way you choose. It is your taste pallet that counts! So use my ideas to create variations of your own.

Honey Mustard

This is the basic dressing. You can create variations of your own besides the two that follow. Add or detract ingredients depending upon your own taste. You'll need:

Apple cider vinegar (3 tablespoons)

Honey mustard (3 tablespoons)

Shake together and drizzle or dump and toss. This dressing goes well on all kinds of greens or greens with legumes. It also tastes great on chicken and fish!

Honey Sweet Hot Mustard

You will need:

Apple cider vinegar (6 tablespoons)

Sweet hot mustard (3 tablespoons)

Honey mustard (3 tablespoons)

Shake ingredients together and either drizzle on your salad or dump and toss. This dressing goes well on all kinds of greens or greens with legumes. It also tastes great on chicken and fish!

Balsamic Honey Mustard

You'll need these ingredients:

Apple cider vinegar (3 tablespoons)

Balsamic vinegar (3 table spoons)

Honey mustard (6 tablespoons)

Shake ingredients together and drizzle over your salad or dump it and toss. Enjoy!

Honey, Lime Juice & Mint

This oil free salad dressing is designed for a nice fruit salad. Choose any kind of fruit (especially berries) and poor or drizle this dressing on and enjoy an eating extravaganza!

You'll need:

1/2 cup of wild honey

1 lime

Fresh organic mint

Squeeze the lime into the 1/2 cup of wild honey, add some mint (about a 1/2 teaspoon) and mix. Then drizzle or dump and toss. You can increase the amount of dressing to fit your needs.

Lime Juice & Ketchup

This one is super easy too! All you need is:

8 limes

2 tables spoons of ketchup

Just shake this concoction in a shaker, drizzle or poor over and toss a salad made of cucumber, tomato, celery, onion (and anything else you want like legumes, fish, shrimp etc) and you have a tasty salad! You can use this dressing to make Ceviche!

Chicken Vegetable Soup That Is Simply Delicious!

I created a chicken vegetable soup that was so lip smacking good that I just have to share it. It should be completely safe because it is made with nothing that is unsafe for those of us who suffer with chronic pancreatitis. The picture is NOT my soup. I am one of the very few people on the planet that does not have a cell phone with a camera or a camera I could use to take digital pictures. So I apologize but I'm serious ...

This chicken vegetable soup is so good you may never make any other kind of chicken vegetable soup. The broth is delightfully sweet (not over sweet, just a hint of sweetness), the soup itself boasts a filling four servings of chicken breast pieces (skinless chicken breasts) and large chunks of vegetables. It will satisfy even the heartiest man sized appetites and is full of protein, vitamins and minerals.

You can create any variations you wish using this recipe for chicken vegetable soup however; adding or subtracting ingredients will obviously change the flavor of the soup so give this specific recipe a try before you create variations. You'll like it.

One of the things you need to remember about me is that I do NOT measure. I am a dumper or a do-it-to-my-taste kinda guy. So I'll list the ingredients with approximate amounts as a starting point and you'll have to go from there. In other words you have to taste it while cooking to see if you need to add more of anything. Naturally I'm being conservative with the spices because once in you can't take them out but you can always add more to your particular taste.

What you'll need:

1.A large pot (5 quarts) with cover

2. 4 Yukon Gold potatoes

3. 6 good sized carrots

4. 3 large parsnips

5. 5 celery stocks

6. Celery leaves (about half a cup)

7. One large yellow onion

8. Salt (1/2 teaspoon)

9. Pepper (1/2 teaspoon)

10. Bay leaves (2 or 3)

11. Basil (1/2 teaspoon)

12. Parsley (1 teaspoon)

13. Garlic (4 – 6 fresh crushed or 1 teaspoon of garlic powder)

14. Thyme (1/4 teaspoon)

Cut up two fresh, skinless chicken breasts (more if you like) and add the chunks to about 3 cups of water (it looked like about 3 cups, maybe it was 4 lol). My pot was about half full of water before I added the chicken. Bring to a boil on high heat and once boiling back down the heat until you have a gentle boil. Cover the pot and cook the chicken for 30 minutes.

While the chicken is cooking wash, peel and cut your vegetables into nice, good sized chunks. And at the 30 minute cooking mark add ALL the vegetables and spices then cook for another 30 minutes or until the vegetables are to your liking for tenderness. Make sure you taste the soup and see if it is to your liking as far as spices. If it needs more ofsome spice add to taste. Once you have the soup broth to your taste liking set the soup aside to "rest" for 10 minutes and then dig in!

Split Pea Soup Is Pancreas Friendly

Split pea soup is one of my favorite soups. I can eat it any time of year in fact I just made a batch so I could write this recipe. Remember I usually "dump" and never measure so it is hard for me to say exactly how I make foods.

But in order to share with you what I eat in order to keep my pancreas from being unhappy I am starting to write down recipes for foods like split pea soup. By the way ... Split pea soup is a wonderful rst solid food to eat after coming out of an acute pancreatitis attack or with symptomatic chronic pancreatitis (after the fast and juice phase) and starting out on what are usually safe solid foods again.

One of the benets of split pea soup is the protein content. According to the package of the peas I use there is 11 grams of protein in a 1/4 cup of split peas.

Green peas are extremely low in fat and a mega source of vitamin K, manganese, ber, B1, copper, folate, phosphorus and vitamin C. Peas also contain a unique assortment phytonutrients that can lower inammation (yep like in the pancreas) and the risk of cancer,

According to this site I use to check out food nutrition there is 16 grams of protein per cooked cup plus a ton of other nutrients. When I look up split pea soup on the same site I nd that there is 10 grams of protein per cup of soup. So I gure my soup is going to boast about the same protein and nutrition content.

Most soup recipes (including pea soup) you'll read about in cookbooks, online or on can and box labels will include oil of some kind. Of course for those who have recurring acute pancreatitis (do to an underlying condition), chronic pancreatitis or sphincter of oddi dysfunction oil (pure fat) is not a good thing.

In order to avoid oil and other high fat ingredients often included in food recipes we, as pancreatitis patients, need to improvise, adapt, overcome. That is often easier said than done and I have found the best way is to simply cook at home, writing, or making up your own recipes.

Let's Make Split Pea Soup!

First we are going to make my basic split pea soup. Underneath the basic version I'll give you other ingredients you can add in order to make variations. Note that making the variations will often change the avor to something more atuned to a vegetable soup with a split pea base.

Ingredients you'll need:

1 pound bag of split peas

1 quart Swanson's Organic Vegetable Broth NOTE: If you are a celiac like me you may not want to use this broth because it contains wheat!

Supposedly the wheat has been processed in some manner to conform to FDA "gluten free" standards. I choose to make my own vegetable broth which is a pain but necessary for my health.

2 nice big onions (chopped or diced)

2 – 3 green onions (chop them all with the green tops)

2 yukon gold potatoes (chopped or diced)

3 medium carrots (diced)

3 stalks of celery with leaves (chopped)

4 cloves of garlic (pressed) or 1 tsp of garlic powder (add more if you like)

1/4 tsp thyme

2 nice bay leaves

1 tsp of black pepper

1 tsp salt (or to taste)

1 tbsp of dried parsley

Directions:

1. Empty the pound of split peas into a 5 quart pan. Put them under the faucet (running almost hot water) and rinse the peas thoroughly swishing the peas with your hand. Pour o water (will be a soapy looking water) being careful not to pour out the peas. Repeat until the water runs clear.

2. Once the water is clear and the peas are clean ll the pan with water until there is about one inch of water above the peas. Set it on the stove (high heat) and bring to a boil. Once peas come to a boil, stir them and make sure none are sticking to the bottom of the pan, then decrease heat to medium and continue to slowly boil the peas for about an hour or until they begin to turn into soup. Do NOT add

ANYTHING until the peas are breaking down. Just peas and water. You might have to add some water so keep your eye on the peas you do not want them to burn!

3. Once the peas have begun to break down add the potatoes, the carrots, the celery, the onions and simmer for another 15 minutes. Stir up nicely. Watch the peas, don't let them burn.

4. Add the vegetable broth and spices and then simmer for another 15 minutes. Stir the soup and check to see if it looks like soup.

5. Check the peas and veggies for tenderness.

6. When the soup looks like this in the pan it is ready to serve

7. Dish your soup up and cover the top in green onion!

8. EAT!

Variations: Making variations to the above soup is simple. Just add extra vegetable ingredients. You can add:

1. Corn (frozen or fresh) which supplies more protein and other nutrients

2. Green peas (frozen or fresh) for more protein, a sweeter taste and more nutrients

3. Spinach (frozen or fresh) for more protein and tons of killer nutrients

4. Green beans (frozen or fresh) for a distinctive green bean avor and nutrition

5. Lima beans (frozen) for more protein and nutrition

You can add one of the above, several or all. Adding other vegetables (you can add almost anything) does change the avor.

Each new vegetable adds

it's own taste and nutrition. Experiment. Have fun and enjoy eating safe split pea soup.

LOW Fat Hot Cocoa (chocolate)

How would you like a nice cup of LOW Fat Hot Cocoa? You know, hot chocolate!

When the chill is in the air something chocolate, cooking on the stove can smell, well, delicious and ... On winter evenings there is nothing like a good cup of hot chocolate!

For those who have pancratitis, can tolerate no fat milk and love chocolate this is a way to get that chocolate x you crave.

Pancreas Friendly LOW Fat Hot Cocoa (chocolate)

Before you try making low fat hot cocoa I'd suggest making sure your pancreas tolerates no fat milk. Some people do, some people don't. I can tolerate some every now and then but denitely not every day. So test no fat milk rst then try this low fat hot chocolate!

Here's how to make homemade hot choclate that actually tastes pretty darn good and has very little fat!

Ingredients you need:

1/2 cup sugar

1/4 cup HERSHEY'S Cocoa (2 grams of fat)

3/4 teaspoon ALCOHOL FREE vanilla extract

4 cups (1 qt.) NO FAT milk

1/3 cup hot water

Marshmallows (if desired)

Directions

1. Stir together sugar, cocoa and salt in medium saucepan; stir in water. Cook over medium heat, stirring constantly, until mixture comes to a boil. Boil and stir 2 minutes. Add milk; stirring constantly, heat to serving temperature. Do Not Boil.

2. Remove from heat; add vanilla. Beat with rotary beater or whisk until foamy. Serve topped with marshmallows, if desired. Five 8-oz. servings.

Dark Chocolate Variation:

RICH, Dark LOW Fat Hot Cocoa (chocolate)

Same as above but add an additional 2Tbsp of Hershey's Special Dark

Cocoa (1 gram of fat)

Whether you tolerate no fat milk or not you'll have to nd out if you want a cup of hot chocolate. As you'll note this makes about a quart of hot chocolate (about 5 cups) so each cup has LESS than 1 gram of fat as far as I can gure.

If you only drink one cup (suggested) save the rest in the pan, put it in the fridge and re-warm it later or drink it as chocolate milk lol

Good luck, hope it works and you like it!

More Variations:

SPICED COCOA: ADD 1/8 teaspoon ground cinnamon and 1/8 teaspoon

ground nutmeg. Serve with cinnamon stick, if desired.

SWISS MOCHA: ADD 2 to 2-1/2 teaspoons powdered instant coee.

CANADIAN COCOA: ADD 1 – 2 teaspoons of pure maple syrup.

MICROWAVE SINGLE SERVING: Combine 1 heaping teaspoon HERSHEY'S

Cocoa, 2 heaping teaspoons sugar and dash salt in microwave-safe cup or mug. Add 2 teaspoons cold milk; stir until smooth. Fill cup with milk.

Microwave at HIGH (100%) 1 to 1-1/2 minutes or until hot. Stir to blend; serve.

Vegetable Broth Recipe

I'm going to give you another of my secret weapons. A food for pancreatitis that I still use to this day, my special pancreatitis vegetable broth. This broth can be used anytime. It is especially good for those just coming out of an acute pancreatitis attack or if you are still suffering pain and nausea from chronic pancreatitis.

I know that I have recommended fresh organic vegetable juice or low sodium V8 juice. The fresh organic vegetable juice made from tomato, carrot, spinach, broccoli, celery, onion and garlic is hard to beat and is much better than this broth but ...

What do you do if you don't have a juicer?

You either buy a juicer so you can juice organic vegetables or you buy low sodium V8 juice. Unfortunately the V8 juice has been processed so much there is very little nutrient value. V8 juice is rich in potassium but lacks in everything else.

Pancreatitis Vegetable Broth Recipe

This is not a fancy recipe and I'm not a chef so don't expect a miraculous, mouth-watering delicacy. It's just a vegetable broth that your inamed pancreas should easily tolerate and will be far superior in nutrients than V8 juice. Be sure to use ORGANIC vegetables for your pancreatitis vegetable broth.

2 tomatoes

2 potatoes

2 carrots

1 cup of sliced celery

1 cup of chopped broccoli

1 cup of scrunched up spinach leaves

1/2 cup of sliced onion

1 clove of fresh garlic (smashed)

Salt and pepper to taste

Make sure everything was washed good before preparation. Cut the stem out of the tomatoes, put them in a pot and then crush them. Next peel the potatoes, set the potatoes aside and put the skins in a pot . Peel the carrots and put the skins in the pot and save the carrots with the potatoes.

Put them into a bowl that will be large enough to hold all the vegetables you are putting into the pot (you remove the potato and carrot skins later and keep the rest).

Throw all the other ingredients into the pot and add enough water to cover the vegetables. If you want a bigger pot of broth just use more vegetables. Turn heat up and watch for the water to steam. NOT BOIL just steam.

Check the temp with a gauge. You want it at 180/190. Just under boiling.

Cover the pot and simmer at that temp for about 10 minutes to kill any bugs (E coli, norovirus, salmonella). Then turn the heat o and let the vegetable broth steep for another 5 – 10 minutes. This leaches the vitamins and minerals from the potato and carrot skins and the other veggies.

Now get a strainer and strain the broth so you have nothing but a nice vegetable broth. Viola you have my pancreatitis vegetable broth. Salt and pepper to taste and drink up.

You can also use it to make vegetable soups etc. Just remember the more you cook stu the less nutrient value it retains because heat kills live enzymes, vitamins, antioxidants, phytonutrients and a lot of minerals. Remove the skins and keep the other veggies. You can now freeze the leftover veggies, including the peeled potatoes and carrots and use them to make soup or boiled taters, carrots and onions. Nothing but the skins go to waste unless you don't like soup or potatoes, carrots and onions.

Give my pancreatitis vegetable broth a try and see how it works for you.

TURKEY TORTELLINI SOUP

INGREDIENTS

- One 12-15 lb. turkey

- 3 medium-size onions

- 6 garlic cloves

- 6 large carrots

- 1 head of celery

- 3 bay leaves

- 6 sprigs fresh thyme

- 1 sprig rosemary

- 3 cups cheese tortellini

- 1 bunch parsley

- ½ cup parmigiano cheese

- ¼ cup extra virgin olive oil

DIRECTIONS:

For Roasting the Turkey

1. Preheat oven to 350°.

2. Place turkey on roasting rack. Season inside and out with salt and pepper.

3. Roast turkey for 2 ½ or 3 hours until internal temperature reaches 155°, basting with natural juices every 30 minutes.

4. Remove turkey and lightly dome with aluminum foil. Allow to cool.

5. Once cool, remove skin and debone turkey.

6. Place body and all bones back into the roasting pan. Roast at 350° for 30 minutes, until bones are dark, golden brown.

7. Shred turkey meat into bite size pieces.

8. Reserve.

For the Turkey Stock

1. In a large stock pot, place turkey bones and body, ½ head of celery (chopped), 3 carrots (chopped), 2 onions (chopped),

4 garlic cloves (smashed), 3 bay leaves, 1 sprig rosemary and 6 sprigs thyme.

2. Cover with 4 inches of water, bring to a simmer.

3. Lower heat and slowly simmer stock for 2 hours, occasionally skimming fat from the top.

4. After 2 hours, strain stock through a fine sift and cheese cloth.

5. Cool and reserve.

For the Garnish

1. Remaining celery, small dice (quarter by quarter inch)

2. Remaining carrots, small dice (quarter by quarter inch)

3. Remaining onions, small dice (quarter by quarter inch)

4. Remaining garlic, minced

5. In a large stock pot, put 2 gallons of water. Add 2 Tbsp. of kosher salt. Bring to a rolling boil and add the tortellini.

6. Cook for 6 minutes, occasionally stirring. Strain.

7. Toss 1 Tbsp. extra virgin olive oil into the tortellini.

8. Lay flat on a sheet tray and allow to cool in refrigerator.

9. Reserve.

To Assemble the Soup

1. Add stock to large stock pot.

2. Add all diced vegetables and bring to a simmer. Cook until carrots are tender, approximately 6-8 minutes.

3. Add shredded turkey meat, tortellini, and finely chopped parsley. Adjust soup seasoning with desired amount of kosher salt and fresh ground pepper.

To Serve

1. In a soup bowl, place 1 large ladle of garnish into center of bowl, top the bowl off with stock.

2. Drizzle with ½ tsp. extra virgin olive oil over the top of the soup.

3. Add 1 Tbsp. of grated parmigiano cheese

Nutritional Data: (assumes 1 oz turkey per bowl) 338 calories,

13 grams fat, 3 grams saturated fat, 39 mg cholesterol, 37 grams carbohydrate, 2.5 grams dietary fiber, 19 grams protein.

TURKEY SWEET POTATO HASH

Since fatigue is sometimes experienced by people living with pancreatic Patients, this easy-to-prepare dish is nutrient dense and a good source of protein and B vitamins, which can help boost energy. In addition, the cooked apple and sweet potato provide fiber that is easily tolerated and full of antioxidants like beta-carotene and quercetin. The ingredients include a variety of appealing textures and flavors of the holiday season! Yield: 6 servings

INGREDIENTS

- 2 medium sweet potatoes, peeled and cut into ½-inch pieces

- 1 medium apple, cored and cut into ½-inch pieces (Honeycrisp or Braeburn work wonderfully, although any apple can suit this recipe)

- ½ cup reduced-fat sour cream (may also substitute reduced-fat yogurt)

- 1 tsp. lemon juice

- 1 Tbsp. olive oil

- 1 medium shallot, chopped

- 3 cups diced, cooked, skinless turkey breast (or chicken)

- 1 tsp. dried rosemary (1 Tbsp. fresh, chopped)

- Salt and pepper, to taste

DIRECTIONS:

1. Place sweet potatoes in a steamer basket and cook for approximately 10 minutes.

Add apple and cook until everything is just tender, about 3 minutes longer.

Be sure that they are not overly mushy. Drain and set aside.

2. Transfer 1 cup of the mixture to a large bowl; mash. Stir in sour cream and lemon juice.

Add the remaining sweet potato/apple mixture and stir gently to mix.

3. Heat oil in a large skillet over medium-high heat. Add shallot until softened, 1 to 2 minutes.

Add turkey (or chicken), rosemary, salt and pepper.

4. Stir mixture occasionally and cook until heated through, about 2 minutes.

5. Add the reserved sweet potato apple mixture to the pan. Press on the hash with a wide

metal spoon or spatula. Cook hash until the bottom is lightly browned, about 3 minutes.

6. Divide into multiple sections with spatula; flip and cook until the bottom sides are browned, about 2 to 3 minutes.

7. Serve promptly

Nutritional Data: 174 calories, 6 grams fat, 2 grams saturated fat,

38 mg cholesterol, 17 grams carbohydrate, 2 grams dietary fiber, 14 grams protein.

SALMON BURGER WITH BOK CHOY, GINGER AND LEMONGRASS

Salmon burgers provide a tasty alternative to old-fashioned beef burgers along with the benefit of healthy omega-3 fats. These burgers have a refreshing appeal from the lemongrass and ginger. Top with traditional plant-based burger toppings on a hearty whole-grain roll. Tuna can be substituted for salmon as well. For those sensitive to spices, they can be toned down as needed. Yield: 4 Servings

INGREDIENTS:

- 1 lb. salmon fillet (or canned salmon)

- 3 cups bok choy, chopped finely (green leafy top only)

- 3 scallions, minced

- 1 Tbsp. finely grated ginger (peeled)

- 1 Tbsp. finely grated lemongrass (dried lemongrass can be substituted if fresh is not found)

- Salt and pepper to taste

- 1 large egg white

- 1 Tbsp. soy sauce

- Cilantro (optional)

DIRECTIONS:

1. Cut salmon into 1/4 inch dice (or use canned salmon), stir into mixture of bok choy, scallions, ginger, lemongrass, salt and pepper in large bowl until combined.

2. Beat together egg white and soy sauce in a small bowl and stir into salmon mixture.

3. Form into four patties that are 1/2 inch thick.

4. Heat non-stick skillet over medium heat. Add 1 Tbsp. of olive oil to cover bottom of skillet. Add salmon patties, cooking for approximately 3-4 minutes per side.

5. Serve hot.

6. Top with cilantro leaves, if desired.

NUTRITIONAL DATA:

173 calories, 7.2 grams fat, 1 gram saturated fat, 50 mg cholesterol, 3.6 grams carbohydrate, 1 gram dietary fiber, 24.3 grams protein

This delicious shrimp dish provides a great source of protein, but can be substituted for chicken for those who may be allergic to shellfish. Tomato content can be reduced to a smaller quantity of diced tomato or omitted and replaced with chicken or vegetable broth in order to reduce acid content. In addition, herbs and spices can be adapted to suit flavor preferences and digestive tolerance. For those looking to add more dietary fiber, whole wheat pasta can be substituted. For those who are experiencing fat malabsorption or dairy intolerance, olive oil can be reduced and parmigiano cheese can be omitted. Yield: 6 Servings

INGREDIENTS:

• 1 lb. angel hair pasta

• 6 Tbsp. extra virgin olive oil

• 3 sprigs fresh thyme

• 8 cloves garlic (sliced paper thin)

• 3/4 cup finely chopped onion

• 1 cup tomato concasse (peeled, seeds removed, diced)

• 1 Tbsp. tomato paste

- 1/2 cup white wine* (can substitute non-alcoholic cooking wine)

- 2 Tbsp. chiffonade fresh basil

(stacked basil leaves, tightly rolled, thinly sliced)

- 3 Tbsp. crushed red pepper flakes** (optional)

- 1 1/2 lb. size 16/20 wild shrimp

- Kosher salt (as needed)

- Fresh ground pepper (as needed)

- 1 Tbsp. minced Italian parsley

- 4 Tbsp. parmigiano cheese (optional)

DIRECTIONS FOR SAUCE:

1. In a medium sized sauce pan add 3 Tbsp. of extra virgin olive oil over medium heat and add onions. Sweat onions for 5 minutes until translucent, then add half the amount of garlic, red pepper flakes (if wanted), 2 sprigs of thyme and tomato paste.

2. Continue to cook over medium heat for 3 minutes. Add white wine (reserving 1 Tbsp. for shrimp).

3. Continue to stir and cook until wine is evaporated. Add tomato concasse, 1 tsp. kosher salt and desired amount of fresh ground pepper. Lower heat to slow simmer for 45 minutes.

4. After 45 minutes, with a hand blender, pulse to slightly puree (you do not want the sauce to be completely smooth). Pulses should be 15 2-second pulses.

5. Add parsley. Reserve for plating.

DIRECTIONS FOR SHRIMP:

1. In a medium sauté pan that's been pre-heated over medium-high heat, add the remaining olive oil and garlic.

2. When the garlic begins to slightly brown, add shrimp that has been shelled and de-veined, season with salt and pepper. Sauté for 1-2 minutes over high heat.

3. Add remaining fresh thyme and 1 Tbsp of white wine. Remove from heat.

4. Reserve for plate assembly.

DIRECTIONS FOR PASTA:

1. In a large stock pot add 2 gallons of water and 3 Tbsp. kosher salt; bring to a boil.

Add angel hair pasta and boil for 3 minutes, achieving doneness of al dente.

2. Strain pasta and put pasta back into pot. Add 3/4 cup tomato sauce to coat pasta.

METHOD FOR ASSEMBLY:

1. Heat shrimp in remaining tomato sauce.

Place desired amount of pasta into a pasta bowl.

2. Spoon over tomato sauce. Add desired amount of shrimp and fresh basil. Each dish can be garnished with 1 Tbsp. parmigiano cheese.

NUTRITIONAL DATA:

497 calories, 17.8 grams fat, 3.4 grams saturated fat, 189 mg cholesterol, 49.3 grams carbohydrate,

1.8 grams dietary fiber, 34 grams protein

SUMMER VEGETABLES OMELET

This omelet is an excellent source of protein and includes squash, which is generally a well-tolerated vegetable. Cheddar cheese can be substituted for another flavor of cheese, or lactose free cheese for those who are lactose intolerant. Yield: Two 2-egg omelets

INGREDIENTS:

- 2/3 cup sliced summer squash

- 2/3 cup sliced fresh zucchini

- 2 Tbsp. oil, divided

- 4 eggs, beaten, divided (may substitute 2 egg whites for each egg if needed for lower fat intake)

- 2 slices white cheddar cheese (use reduced fat cheese if experiencing fat intolerance or any flavor cheese of choice)

DIRECTIONS:

1. Heat 1 Tbsp. oil in omelet pan over medium heat.

2. Sauté zucchini and squash in oil for 4-5 minutes until tender.

3. Remove vegetables and keep warm.

4. Add additional Tbsp. oil to warm pan. Add two beaten eggs and half of the vegetables. Flip and cook thoroughly. Fold in half and top with 1 slice of white cheddar cheese.

5. Make second omelet with remaining ingredients.

NUTRITIONAL DATA:

310 calories, 27.4 grams fat, 9.1 grams saturated fat, 193 mg cholesterol, 3.6 grams carbohydrate, 0.8 grams dietary fiber, 13.4 grams protein

CHICKEN SALAD SANDWICH

This sandwich is very easy to prepare and contains satisfying flavors and textures. It is a well-balanced meal that includes protein and carbohydrates, along with a splash of colorful fruit and herbs. For those experiencing fat intolerance, reduced fat mayo can be substituted and walnuts can be avoided. You can also experiment with other herbs like rosemary or basil for varied flavors. Yield: 4 sandwiches

INGREDIENTS:

• 2 chicken breasts (skin on during cooking only) or approximately

2 cups diced or shredded cooked, skinless chicken

• 2 Tbsp. mayonnaise (may substitute yogurt - low fat or Greek - and 1 tsp. lemon juice)

• 1/4 cup sliced grapes

- 2 Tbsp. dried cranberries

- 1/4 cup chopped walnuts (optional)

- 2 tsp. dried tarragon

- 8 slices bread

DIRECTIONS:

1. Preheat oven to 375°.

2. Roast chicken breasts for approximately 45 minutes until cooked through, juices run clear and temperature of chicken reaches 165°.

3. Remove skin from breast meat. Discard skin. Cube, dice, or shred meat.

4. Add mayonnaise, grapes, cranberries, walnuts, and tarragon.

5. Mix well and divide into 4 (~3/4 cup) portions and spread onto bread.

Delicious with toasted bread!

NUTRITIONAL DATA:

237 calories, 9.8 grams fat, 1.4 grams saturated fat, 56 mg cholesterol, 13.1 grams carbohydrate, 1.2 grams dietary fiber, 23.7 grams protein

CHICKEN KEBAB WITH TZATZIKI AND PITA

A great summer time chicken recipe topped with cool, creamy tzatziki sauce. Preparation is required 2-3 hours ahead of time but well worth the extra wait time. Choose this recipe for those needing high protein, low fiber choices. Yield: 6 servings

INGREDIENTS:

Pita:

• 1 pack store-bought pita bread Tzatziki sauce:

• 3 cucumbers

• 12 oz. plain Greek yogurt

• 1 pinch of sea salt

• 1/2 tsp. extra virgin olive oil

• 2 cloves of garlic, minced

Chicken:

- 1 1/2 pounds skinless, boneless chicken breast halves, cut into 1/2 inch pieces

- 1/4 cup olive oil for marinade

- 2 Tbsp. lemon juice

- 1 tsp. dried oregano

- 1/2 tsp. sea salt

- 6 wooden skewers

DIRECTIONS:

Tzatziki sauce:

1. Clean and grate cucumbers. Be sure to remove seeds and peel off cucumber skin if on a low-fiber diet.

2. Strain juice and place in medium bowl.

3. Add yogurt to bowl and mix cucumbers, garlic, salt and olive oil together.

4. Cover and refrigerate for 30 minutes.

Chicken and pita:

1. Combine 1/4 cup olive oil, lemon juice, 1 tsp. oregano, and 1/2 tsp. sea salt in a large bowl.

2. Add chicken, mix with the marinade and cover the bowl.

3. Marinate in the refrigerator for at least 2 hours.

4. Skewer chicken evenly on 6 wooden skewers.

Preheat grill, place pitas on grill for 2 minutes on each side until slightly browned.

5. Remove from grill and set aside.

6. Cook the skewers on the preheated grill, turning frequently until nicely browned on all sides, about 10 minutes per side. Serve with grilled pita and topped with tzatziki sauce

NUTRITIONAL DATA:

441 calories, 13.8 grams fat, 3 grams saturated fat, 67 mg cholesterol, 44.7 grams carbohydrate, 3 grams dietary fiber, 34.9 grams protein

EDAMAME HUMMUS WRAP

Soy is a high-quality protein that does not cause the same discomfort that other beans and hummuses can. This recipe is extremely easy and satisfying. Can be delicious plain or with any added vegetables that you can tolerate (those with diarrhea or indigestion should be sure to use well-cooked vegetables without the skin). Yield: 4 servings

INGREDIENTS:

- 1 cup cooked shelled edamame

- 1/4 cup Tahini (sesame paste)

- 1 Tbsp. lemon juice

- Garlic clove, peeled

- 2 Tbsp. coarsely chopped fresh herbs (such as rosemary, thyme, and basil)

- 2 Tbsp. olive oil

- Salt to taste (approximately 1/4 tsp.)

- 4 flour wraps

- Optional: Sautéed or roasted vegetables, or fresh, raw vegetables that you can tolerate

DIRECTIONS:

1. Combine edamame, tahini, lemon juice, garlic, and herbs in food processor.

2. Process ingredients until smooth.

3. Drizzle olive oil through feed tube of food processor, continuing to process until the oil is fully incorporated into the hummus mixture.

4. Season with salt to taste.

5. Spread 1/4 cup hummus in each wrap, top with raw or roasted vegetables of choice, roll and serve.

NUTRITIONAL DATA:

399 calories, 21.9 grams fat, 3.1 grams saturated fat, 0 mg cholesterol, 39.9 grams carbohydrate, 4.1 grams dietary fiber, 12.1 grams protein

CHICKEN WITH QUINOA

Prepared as described this recipe will "pack a protein punch", but for additional protein add white beans and cook the quinoa in chicken broth. To add additional flavor or variety, top with low-fat sour cream and salsa for a Mexican-inspired dish. Other grains such as bulgur, rice, or couscous can also be used. Yield: 6 servings

INGREDIENTS:

- 1 Tbsp. olive oil, divided
- 1 lb. ground chicken breast
- 1 tsp. rosemary
- Pinch salt (optional)
- 1/4 tsp. pepper (optional)
- 1 cup quinoa
- 1 1/2 cups frozen kale
- 1/4 cup chicken broth

DIRECTIONS:

1. Heat 2 tsp. olive oil in skillet; add the ground chicken, rosemary, salt, and pepper.

2. Cook until cooked through and browned.

3. Add frozen kale and chicken broth and allow to thaw and wilt; approximately 2-3 minutes.

4. While the chicken is cooking, separately cook quinoa according to package directions in medium size saucepan

with remaining tsp. of olive oil. Fluff with fork when cooked.

5. Add quinoa to skillet with chicken and kale and combine well. Serve warm.

NUTRITIONAL DATA:

217 calories, 4.8 grams fat, 0.6 grams saturated fat, 47 mg cholesterol, 19.9 grams carbohydrate, 2.8 grams dietary fiber, 23.9 grams protein

VEGETABLE POPOVER

These vegetable popovers are excellent for individuals needing soft, easy-to-swallow foods. Eggs (or egg substitute) add an excellent source of high-quality protein. This is also a great recipe to prepare ahead of time and reheat as a healthy mini-meal. Yield: 6 servings

INGREDIENTS:

• 1 zucchini, chopped into bite-size pieces

• 1 large carrot, chopped into small pieces (about half the size of the zucchini)

- 2 tsp. olive oil

- 6 large eggs

- 1/4 cup milk (non-dairy alternative, if desired)

- 1/3 cup shredded cheddar cheese (use reduced-fat cheese for those experiencing fat intolerance)

- Salt and freshly ground black pepper, to taste

- Pinch of turmeric

- Onion powder, to taste

DIRECTIONS:

1. Preheat the oven to 350°.

2. Spray 6 muffin cups with nonstick spray.

3. Sauté the zucchini and the carrots in 2 tsp. olive oil for 5-7 minutes.

4. In a medium bowl, whisk together the eggs and milk. Add salt, pepper, turmeric, and onion powder.

5. Distribute egg mixture evenly into muffin cups.

6. Distribute zucchini and carrots into egg mixture.

7. Bake 25 to 30 minutes, or until egg is cooked through.

NUTRITIONAL DATA:

Nutritional Data: 126 calories, 8.9 grams fat, 3.2 grams saturated fat, 193 mg cholesterol, 3.4 grams carbohydrate, 0.7 grams dietary fiber, 8.7 grams protein

ASPARAGUS FRITTATA

Frittatas are very versatile – they can be used at any meal as a main dish, side dish or appetizer, and can easily be turned into a quiche by adding a pie crust at the bottom (if able to tolerate higher amounts of fat). Eggs provide the highest quality protein available in any food. This recipe is great for those needing easy to chew/swallowing foods. Yield: 1 9-inch quiche, serves 6

NUTRITIONAL DATA:

125 calories, 8.8 grams fat, 4.6 grams saturated fat, 127 mg cholesterol, 2.2 grams carbohydrate, 0.9 grams dietary fiber, 9.9 grams protein

INGREDIENTS:

• 1/2 lb. fresh asparagus, trimmed and cut into 1/2 inch pieces

• 1 egg white, lightly beaten

- 4 eggs, beaten

- 1 1/2 cups fat-free or low-fat milk

- 1/4 tsp. ground nutmeg

- 1 Tbsp. Dijon mustard

- 1 cup shredded Swiss or muenster cheese (use reduced fat cheese if experiencing fat intolerance)

- Salt and pepper to taste

DIRECTIONS:

1. Preheat oven to 375°.

2. Add asparagus to saucepan with 1 inch of water or place in a steamer. Steam for 4-6 minutes or until tender but not mushy. Once steamed, allow it to drain well and cool.

3. Coat pie dish with nonstick cooking spray.

4. Add drained and dried asparagus to pie dish.

5. In a bowl, beat together eggs, milk, mustard, nutmeg, salt and pepper. Add shredded cheese and mix in.

6. Pour egg mixture into pie pan.

7. Bake uncovered in preheated oven until firm, about 40-50 minutes.

8. Enjoy warm or at room temperature.

NUTRITIONAL DATA:

125 calories, 8.8 grams fat, 4.6 grams saturated fat, 127 mg cholesterol, 2.2 grams carbohydrate, 0.9 grams dietary fiber, 9.9 grams protein

PUMPKIN OATMEAL BARS

These are a healthy alternative to many common cookie recipes. Whole-wheat flour, oats, pumpkin, and ground flaxseed add soluble and insoluble fiber, along with the phytochemical and antioxidant benefits of the added spices. Great selections for an after dinner dessert or midday snack. Flaxseed can be omitted if experiencing gas, bloating, or diarrhea. Yield: 40 square bars or 48 cookies

INGREDIENTS:

• 2 cups whole-wheat flour

• 1 1/3 cups rolled oats

• 1 tsp. baking soda

- 3/4 tsp. salt

- 1 tsp. cinnamon

- 1/2 tsp. nutmeg

- 1 1/3 cup sugar

- 2/3 cup canola oil

- 3 Tbsp. molasses

- 1 can of cooked pumpkin puree

- 1 tsp. vanilla

- 2 Tbsp. ground flaxseed (optional)

- Optional add-ins: 1 cup mini chocolate chips

DIRECTIONS:

1. Preheat oven to 350°. Grease two 12 x 17 baking sheet pans.

2. Mix together flour, oats, baking soda, salt, and spices.

3. In a separate bowl, mix together sugar, oil, molasses, pumpkin, vanilla, and optional flaxseeds until very well combined.

4. Mix flour and sugar mixtures together. Fold in chocolate chips, if desired.

5. Spread and press batter onto greased cookie sheets (to make cookies, drop 1 inch size balls of batter an inch apart, and flatten tops of cookies with fork or your fingers to press into cookie shape).

6. Bake for 16 minutes or until inserted knife or toothpick is clean. Rotate halfway through baking.

7. Remove from oven (if making cookies, transfer to wire rack to cool).

8. Once cool slice into 20 bars per sheet pan.

NUTRITIONAL DATA:

101 calories, 4 grams fat, 0 grams saturated fat, 0 mg cholesterol, 15.4 grams carbohydrate, 0.9 grams dietary fiber, 1.2 grams protein

BAKED BERRY FRENCH TOAST

This French toast recipe is great to make ahead of time for a busy weekday morning. It is a good balanced entrée that includes protein, carbohydrates, dairy, and fruit. Cream cheese and milk components can be substituted with lactose-free versions for those experiencing lactose intolerance. Yield: 8 Servings

INGREDIENTS:

• 12 slices day-old bread, cut into

1-inch cubes

• 1 (12 oz.) package of low-fat cream cheese, room temperature

• 2 1/4 cups low-fat fat-free milk or non-dairy alternative, divided

• 2 tsp. vanilla, divided

• 2 cups blueberries, fresh or thawed frozen, divided

• 10 eggs, beaten

• 1/4 cup plus 1 Tbsp. honey or pure maple syrup

DIRECTIONS:

1. Preheat oven to 350°.

2. Lightly grease a 9x13 inch-baking dish.

3. Blend 1 brick of cream cheese, 1/4 cup of milk, 1 Tbsp. honey and 1 tsp. vanilla.

4. Arrange 1/2 of the bread cubes in bottom of dish. Top with cream cheese mixture.

Sprinkle 1 cup of blueberries over top, and top with remaining bread cubes.

5. In large bowl, mix eggs, milk, vanilla extract, and honey or syrup. Pour over bread cubes Cover, refrigerate 1 hour or overnight.

6. Cover, and bake for 30 minutes. Uncover, and continue baking for 25-30 minutes, until center is firm and surface is lightly browned.

7. Let cool for 10-12 minutes. Top with remaining berries and enjoy.

NUTRITIONAL DATA:

231 calories, 7.5 grams fat, 1.7 grams saturated fat, 205 mg cholesterol, 29 grams carbohydrate, 3.8 grams dietary fiber, 13.7 grams protein

BANANA BLUEBERRY MUFFINS

These muffins are a great quick breakfast treat, with bananas and blueberries providing soluble fiber, potassium, and phytonutrients. Non-dairy milk can be substituted for those who are intolerant to lactose and whole-wheat flour can be substituted to increase the fiber content. Yield: 12 muffins

INGREDIENTS:

- 1/2 cup mashed ripe banana (about 1 large)

- 1/2 cup granulated sugar

- 1/2 cup milk (may also sub any non-dairy milk)

- 1/3 cup canola oil

- 1 Tbsp. vanilla extract

- 1 tsp. cinnamon

- 1 cup all-purpose flour (or whole wheat flour)

- 2 tsp. baking powder

- 1/2 cup frozen blueberries

DIRECTIONS:

1. Preheat oven to 400°.

2. Line muffin pan with paper cups.

3. In a large bowl, mash the banana with a fork.

4. Add the sugar, milk, oil, vanilla, cinnamon, and whisk until combined.

5. Add the flour, baking powder, and stir until just combined; don't over mix.

6. Fold in 1/2 cup frozen blueberries.

7. Add batter to muffin tin (for easy distribution use medium cookie scoop)

8. Bake for 15-20 minutes, or until tops are slightly golden.

NUTRITIONAL DATA:

Nutritional Data: 125 calories, 6.4 grams fat, 0.6 grams saturated fat, 1 mg cholesterol, 15.5 grams carbohydrate, 0.7 grams dietary fiber, 1.5 grams protein

CARROT PURÉE WITH OLIVE OIL AND CILANTRO

This is the perfect side dish for the holiday season, especially for patients facing pancreatic cancer, as it is a well-cooked vegetable dish which is easier to digest and less likely to aggravate digestive issues. The carrots provide an excellent source of beta-carotene. The oil may be reduced if sensitive to fat, or coconut oil may be substituted (which may be more easily absorbed). If you are sensitive to additional herbed flavors, the cilantro can be reduced or omitted. This purée can also translate well to any other root vegetable or squash – such as turnip, parsnip, acorn squash, or butternut squash. Yield: 6 servings

INGREDIENTS:

• About 10 carrots, peeled and cubed

• 5 Tbsp. extra virgin olive oil

• Sea salt

• Fresh black pepper

• 3 Tbsp. finely chopped fresh cilantro (may substitute other fresh herbs of choice and as tolerated)

DIRECTIONS:

1. In a large pot, boil peeled and cubed carrots for about 20 minutes until they are very tender. (Alternatively, steaming them in a steam pan over boiling water may preserve the maximum amount of nutrients.)

2. In a medium pan, add fresh cilantro leaves and 3 Tbsp. of extra virgin olive oil. Heat on lowest flame for about 5 minutes.

3. Remove from heat and allow to sit for about 5 minutes. Remove cilantro from oil and set aside.

4. In a food processor or using an immersion blender, add in cooked carrots and cilantro oil and 2 Tbsp. of extra virgin olive oil. Purée until smooth.

5. Add sea salt and fresh black pepper to taste and fresh cilantro as a garnish.

NUTRITIONAL DATA:

142 calories, 11.7 grams fat, 1.7 grams saturated fat, 0 mg cholesterol, 10 grams carbohydrate, 2.5 grams dietary fiber, 0.8 grams protein

Cold-Weather Recipes for Pancreatitis Patients

Quick Eight- Vegetable Soup

If you're rushing around this week, dinner may seem like a daunting new task. Don't worry! We have a healthy dish you can prepare in a breeze. Frozen veggies cut down on prep time and thanks to flash-freezing technology, contain the same nutrients as their fresh counterparts. Beans add protein and extra fiber. Serve this soup with some warm, crusty whole grain bread for a quick and wholesome meal.

Ingredients

- 1 Tbsp. extra virgin olive oil
- 1 chopped onion
- 4 cup low-sodium vegetable broth
- 1/2 cup frozen baby lima beans
- 1 (15 oz.) can no salt added back, Great Northern, or navy beans
- 1 cup frozen mixed vegetables
- 1/2 cup frozen tri-colored bell peppers
- 2 tsp. dried oregano or thyme
- Pinch of dried red pepper flakes
- 1 cup frozen broccoli florets
- Salt, to taste
- 1/4 cup grated Parmesan cheese

Makes 4 servings (1 1/3 cup). Per serving: 250 calories, 8 g total fat (2 g saturated fat, 0 g trans fat), 5 mg cholesterol, 32 g carbohydrates, 10 g protein, 9 g dietary fiber, 410 mg sodium, 5 g sugar, 0 g added sugar.

Directions

In a large saucepan, heat oil over medium-high heat. Add onion and cook until translucent, about 5 minutes, stirring occasionally. Add broth and bring liquid to boil. Add lima beans, reduce heat and simmer covered for 5 minutes.

Add canned beans, mixed vegetables, peppers, oregano and pepper flakes and simmer covered for 5 minutes. Add broccoli, cover, and cook for 5 minutes. Add salt to taste. This soup keeps covered in refrigerator for 3 days. Reheat in covered pot over medium heat.

To serve, divide soup among deep bowls. Option to top each serving with 1 tablespoon of Parmesan cheese.

New American Beef Stew

One-pot meals are the original convenience food. They're easy, versatile, and can pack plenty of healthy ingredients. This stew features kale, green beans, carrots and, yes, even beef. That's because even traditional, comforting favorites like beef stew can fit into a healthy lifestyle with a few modifications and proper portion control. Just remember to limit beef and other red meat to no more than 18 cooked ounces per week for a lower cancer risk.

Ingredients

- 2 Tbsp. extra virgin olive oil
- 1 lb lean beef stew meat, cut into 1-inch cubes
- 2 large onions, chopped

- 4 medium carrots, cubed
- 2 cups cups diced leeks, rinsed well
- 6 garlic cloves, finely chopped
- 2 cans (14.5 ounces each) diced tomatoes in juice
- 2 cans (6 ounces each) tomato paste
- 2 cans (14.5 ounces each) fat-free, reduced sodium beef broth
- 3 Tbsp. dried oregano
- 2 cups water
- 2 large potatoes, cubed
- 1 1/4 lbs frozen green beans
- 2 cups chopped kale
- Salt and freshly ground black pepper

Makes 6 servings (1.5 cup). Per serving: 440 calories, 10 g total fat (2.5 g saturated fat, 0 g trans fat), 50 mg cholesterol, 64 g carbohydrates, 29 g protein, 12 g dietary fiber, 350 mg sodium, 20 g sugar, 0 g added sugar.

Directions

In a large pot or stockpot, heat olive oil over medium-high heat.

Add 1/2 of beef and sauté for about 5 minutes, stirring, until browned on all sides. Remove beef from pot and set aside. Repeat procedure with remaining beef.

In the same pot, sauté onions for about 5 minutes, stirring often until translucent. Remove onions from pot and set aside.

Add carrots, leeks, and garlic, and sauté for about 5 minutes, stirring often, until barely tender. Return beef and onions to pot. Add tomatoes with juice, tomato paste, broth, oregano, and water, and bring to a boil. Reduce heat to low and simmer for about 1 hour, until beef is almost tender.

Add potatoes and bring back to a boil. Lower heat, cover partially, and simmer for about 15 minutes, until potatoes are barely tender.

Add green beans and kale and cook for another 6 to 8 minutes, until kale is tender.

Season to taste with salt and pepper and serve.

Sweet Potato Chili with Peanuts

This vegetarian one-pot meal will warm you up on even the coldest of winter days. Earthy sweet potatoes and carrots form the base and provide cancer-fighting fiber and carotenoids. Tomatoes, peppers and onion add even more flavor and nutrition. Ready in just 45 minutes, serve over a whole grain for a balanced, cancer preventive dinner.

Ingredients

- 2 Tbsp. canola oil
- 1 medium onion, chopped
- 2 medium carrots, peeled and thinly sliced
- 1 medium green bell pepper, seeded and chopped
- 1 medium red bell pepper, seeded and chopped
- 3 garlic cloves, minced
- 2 pounds sweet potatoes, peeled and cut into bite-sized chunks (about 4 cups)
- 1 1/2 cups unsalted roasted peanuts
- 1 can (28 ounces) crushed tomatoes in juice
- 1 can (6 ounces) tomato paste
- 2 cans (4 ounces each) diced mild green chiles with liquid
- 4-6 chili powder, to taste
- 1 Tbsp. ground cumin, to taste
- 1 Tbsp. sugar
- Salt and freshly ground pepper, to taste

Makes 10 servings (about 1 cup per serving). Per serving: 310 calories, 15 g total fat (2 g saturated fat, 0 g trans fat), 0 mg cholesterol, 41 g carbohydrates, 11 g protein, 9 g dietary fiber, 470 mg sodium, 15 g sugar, 1 g added sugar.

Directions

In a large, heavy pot, heat the canola oil over medium heat.

Add the onion, carrots, and bell peppers and sauté, stirring occasionally, for about 8 minutes, until vegetables are golden.

Add the garlic and sauté stirring constantly for 30 seconds, until fragrant. Stir in the sweet potatoes, peanuts, tomatoes and juice, tomato paste, chiles and their liquid, chili powder, cumin and sugar.

Bring to a boil, then reduce the heat to low immediately and simmer gently, stirring occasionally, for 15 to 25 minutes until the sweet potatoes are just tender.

Halfway through the cooking process, adjust the seasonings, adding more chili powder and cumin, if desired. Season to taste with salt and pepper and serve.

Pumpkin Mac and Cheese

If you are looking for a unique twist on a classic dish, look no further. This pumpkin mac and cheese is a wonderful way to add a nutritional boost to your usual mac and cheese recipe. Pumpkins are rich in carotenoids, particularly alpha- and beta-carotene, high in fiber and provide 100% of your daily value of vitamin A in just one serving. This creamy, delicious dish is not only perfect for a fall dinner, but contains 14g of protein and 5g of dietary fiber.

Ingredients

- Canola oil cooking spray
- 1/2 cup panko bread crumbs
- 1/3 cup grated Parmesan cheese
- 8 oz. whole-wheat pasta
- 1 cup low-fat (1%) milk
- 1 Tbsp. unsalted butter
- 1 Tbsp. all-purpose flour
- 1 1/2 cups (2 1/2 oz.) sharp light (50 percent) Cheddar cheese
- 1 cup canned unsweetened pumpkin
- 1/2 tsp. mustard powder
- 1/4 tsp. ground black pepper
- Pinch of cayenne pepper
- 1/8 tsp. ground nutmeg, optional

Makes 6 servings. Per serving: 260 calories, 6 g total fat (3 g saturated fat), 38 g carbohydrates, 14 g protein, 6 g dietary fiber, 230 mg sodium, 5 g sugar, 0 g added sugar.

Directions

Preheat oven to 375 degrees F. Coat 6 cup baking dish with cooking spray and set aside.

In a separate bowl mix together breadcrumbs and Parmesan cheese and toss to combine. Set mixture aside.

In large pot, boil 4 quarts of water. Add pasta and cook for 10 minutes, until slightly al dente. Drain in colander, and set aside.

While pasta is cooking, heat milk in microwave or small saucepan, until it steams, and set aside.

In large saucepan, melt butter over medium heat. Whisk in flour and cook for 1 minute, whisking slowly. Remove from heat and gradually add milk while whisking to avoid lumps. Return pot to medium-high heat and simmer sauce until it thickens to consistency of stirred yogurt, about 3 minutes.

Add Cheddar cheese, pumpkin, mustard, black and cayenne peppers and nutmeg (optional), and stir until cheese melts completely.

Mix in cooked pasta to cheese mixture.

Spread mac and cheese in prepared baking dish and sprinkle with breadcrumb and parmesan cheese mixture over top.

Bake 15-20 minutes or until breadcrumbs are crisp and golden brown. Serve immediately.

Pancreatits smoothies recipes

Mango Carrot Ginger Smoothie

Ingredients

- 1 mango, peeled, sliced into chunks
- 1/2 orange, peeled, quartered
- 1 large carrot, sliced into large chunks
- 1 1/2 cups soy milk, plain
- 1 (1-inch) piece, peeled fresh ginger
- 6 ice cubes

Makes 2 servings (1 1/4 cups). Per serving: 190 calories, 4 g total fat (0.5 g saturated fat, 0 g trans fat), 0 mg cholesterol, 36 g carbohydrates, 7 g protein, 3 g dietary fiber, 90 mg sodium, 28 g sugar, 0 g added sugar.

Directions

Place all ingredients in a blender and process until smooth.

Pour into 2 glasses.

Tips

Frozen mango chunks may be used if fresh mango is not available.

Blueberry Blast Smoothie

Ingredients

- 2 cups frozen unsweetened blueberries (do not thaw)
- 1/2 cup orange juice (calcium-fortified preferred)
- 3/4 cup low-fat or nonfat vanilla yogurt
- 1/2 medium frozen banana
- 1/2 tsp. pure vanila extract

Makes 2 servings. Per serving: 220 calories, 2.5 g total fat (1 g saturated fat, 0 g trans fat), 5 mg cholesterol, 46 g carbohydrates, 6 g protein, 5 g dietary fiber, 65 mg sodium, 35 g sugar.

Directions

Place blueberries, orange juice, yogurt, banana and vanilla into blender.

Cover securely and blend for 30 to 35 seconds or until thick and smooth. For thinner smoothies, add more juice; for thicker smoothies, add more frozen fruit.

Pour into 2 glasses and serve immediately.

Tips

Don't have frozen blueberries? Try frozen pineapple, cherries or mango.

Not Your Ordinary Water

The water with fresh strawberries and mint leaves was refreshing and ever so slightly sweet. Here's how to make it:

1. Slice 1/2 cup fresh strawberries

2. Select several sprigs of fresh mint and rinse if needed

Add to 1-2 quarts of fresh, cold water and refrigerate for several hours to let flavors mingle. The longer you let it soak (even up to a day), the more prominent the flavors will become.

The pitcher of lemon and basil water was just as unique and delicious:

1. Slice 1 whole lemon

2. Select 1/4 – 1/2 cup fresh basil leaves

Add to 1-2 quarts of fresh, cold water and refrigerate as in the previous recipe. This water reminded me of a fragrant, summer herb garden.

Flavoring your water with fruits and herbs is a great way to drink more water – you can still get great taste, without the added calories typical of many drinks. Sodas, sports drinks and even fruit juice, can be high in calories and sugar. Too many of these can lead to overweight and obesity (adding 2 cans of coke a day could mean 3 pounds weight gain a month) which increases risk for many common cancers.

Mango Carrot Ginger Smoothie

Ingredients:

- 1 mango, peeled, sliced into chunks
- 1/2 orange, peeled, quartered
- 1 large carrot, sliced into large chunks
- 1-2 cups kale or spinach
- 1 1/2 cups soy milk, plain
- 1 inch piece, peeled fresh ginger
- 6 ice cubes
- Option: Garnish with fresh mint

Makes 2 servings. Per serving: 200 calories, 4 g total fat (0 g. saturated fat), 36 g carbohydrate, 7 g protein, 4 g dietary fiber, 120 mg sodium.

Directions

Place all ingredients in blender and process until smooth.

Pour into 2 glasses. Enjoy!

Peaches & Cream SmoothieFavorite

Simple meals like shakes and smoothies are often helpful ways for people caring for or living with pancreatitis to get the nutrients they need. This Peaches and Cream Smoothie combines the potassium and fiber benefits of peaches and bananas along with soluble fiber from rolled oats, which can help to alleviate loose bowel movements and promote regularity. The protein powder can be added at the recommendation of your healthcare team for additional nutritional value. Dairy components can be easily substituted with lactose-free or non-dairy versions.

Directions

1. Gather all ingredients.

2. Combine ingredients in a blender and enjoy.

3. Store in a container in your refrigerator overnight if making ahead of time. In the morning, add last 1/4 cup milk, more if you need it to blend smoothly.

Best Anti-Inflammatory Smoothie

Are your inflammatory pains and aches getting in your way? Alleviate some of its symptoms with an inflammation-fighting smoothie packed with powerful detoxifying ingredients. This delicious recipe packs a punch of flavors and nutrients to combat inflammation and free radicals that harm the cells in your body. With anti-inflammatory ingredients, like cherries, turmeric, and cinnamon, this smoothie can help you relieve some of the pain that's been holding you back

Ingredients

- 1 cup Lacinto Kale
- 1/2 cup Cherries (pitted)
- 1/2 Banana
- 1 1/2 cup Coconut Water
- 1 tbsp Chia Seeds
- 1 tbsp Ginger Root, fresh
- 1/2 tsp Turmeric, ground
- 1/4 tsp Cinnamon, ground

Directions

1 Add ingredients in the order listed and blend until smooth.

2 Enjoy!

Doctor Designed Anti-Inflammatory and Gut Healing Smoothie

Ingredients

- 1½ cups of unsweetened flax milk
- ½ cup frozen mangos
- ½ cup fresh papaya
- ¼ cups walnuts
- ½ inch fresh ginger root
- ½ inch fresh turmeric root
- ½ teaspoon ground cinnamon
- 1 Tablespoon chia seeds
- 1 Tablespoon flax seeds
- 1 scoop L-glutamine powder*
- ¼ teaspoon probiotic powder*

Preparation

Place the flax milk in the blender first and then add the remaining ingredients. If you have a Vitamix you will not need to grind the nuts or seeds prior. If you do not have a powerful blender, I recommend grinding the nuts and seeds in a coffee grinder before placing them in the blender.

*You can make the smoothie without these if you choose. I personally use them daily in all my smoothies. I also recommend using all organic ingredients if possible.

Makes one large smoothie.

Enjoy!

PEACHES AND CREAM SMOOTHIE
Simple meals like shakes and smoothies are often helpful ways for people caring for or living with pancreatitis to get the nutrients they need. This Peaches and Cream Smoothie combines the potassium and fiber benefits of peaches and bananas along with soluble fiber from rolled oats, which can help to alleviate loose bowel movements and promote regularity. The protein powder can be added at the recommendation of your healthcare team for additional nutritional value. Dairy components can be easily substituted with lactose-free or non-dairy versions. Yield: 1-2 servings

INGREDIENTS:

- ½ cup rolled oats

- cup plain yogurt (or soy/coconut/almond yogurt)

- ¾ cup milk (or soy/almond/rice milk) + ¼ cup more for morning

- 1 small ripe peach (or ½ cup frozen peaches, thawed and softened)

- ½ medium banana

- Pinch of salt

- 1-2 Tbsp. protein powder (whey or soy) (optional)

DIRECTIONS:

1. Gather all ingredients

2. Combine ingredients in a blender and enjoy

3. Store in a container in your refrigerator overnight if making ahead of time. In the morning, add last ¼ cup milk, more if you need it to blend smoothly.

Nutritional Data: (assumes regular whole milk and yogurt)

426 calories, 9 grams fat, 4.5 grams saturated fat,

25 mg cholesterol, 68 grams carbohydrate, 7 grams dietary fiber, 20 grams protein

Made in the USA
Las Vegas, NV
03 May 2024

89492682R00056